For my family and friends: Thank you for your love and support. And to my wife Rian, who makes every day worth living.

Chapter I: Why I Wrote this Book

My first two patients on my internal medicine clerkship died of COVID-19. They may have shared a diagnosis and cause of death, but nothing else about their experiences in life or in death were the same. I will remember each person vividly for the rest of my life.

Mrs. P had just been transferred to our floor from the ICU. We discussed her love of cooking; she had been an elementary school cafeteria chef locally in the Bronx for decades. I also got to know her husband of 25 years, who stood by her side throughout visitor hours, which were limited at the time. A few days later, when I walked into her room, Mrs. P looked down despondently at her bedsheets. I walked over and sat quietly in a chair beside her. After a few moments she looked up, her eyes red and welling with tears. She strained to speak, and I could barely hear her through her oxygen mask.

"Adam, I don't want to die. I don't want to leave my family, but I feel like giving up."

I placed my hand on her shoulder as her words seemed to hang in the air. I thought about all she had been through since admission 3 weeks ago. She'd been placed on a ventilator twice and had come back and forth from the ICU. I sat with her because it was all I could do at the time, and I wanted her to feel the presence of a supportive caretaker by her side. I wanted to acknowledge the terrible trauma she had endured since being in the hospital. I told her she was strong, that I was glad she had not given up and that I was sure many people, including her family and the students at her school, were also grateful.

Despite our best efforts, Mrs. P would go on to die in the ICU ten days later. Her suffering leading up to her death was deeply saddening. I felt helpless, wishing that I had more to offer her to help heal her failing lungs and alleviate her emotional distress. Her death seemed drawn out to me, prolonged and cruel. I wondered at what point, as doctors, we might be doing more harm than good.

That same week, I experienced the death of a patient even more suddenly. I heard a cardiac arrest code and ran to what I immediately realized was my patient's room. Ms. R, a 48-year-old mother of three who I had been following for only a day, was medically stable just a few hours earlier and my team thought she might have her worst COVID-19 days behind her. When I got to the room, I began chest compressions, alternating with the resident until she died. It was surreal and heartbreaking, and unlike Mrs. P, I cannot even recall our last conversation.

I often think about both women and wish things had ended differently. Ultimately, my experiences so close to death have further confirmed my reasons for aspiring to be a doctor.

In the summer of 2021, when I was preparing to apply to residency, I learned that the number of applicants to US MD-granting medical schools had increased from 53,030 in 2020 to 62,443 in 2021.[1] That is nearly an 18% increase in applicants. One might speculate that this is due to students finding their calling to medicine

[1] Weiner, Stacy. "Applications to Medical School Are at an All-Time High. What Does This Mean for Applicants and Schools?" *AAMC*, 22 Oct. 2020, https://www.aamc.org/news-insights/applications-medical-school-are-all-time-high-what-does-mean-applicants-and-schools.

due to the pandemic. Some refer to this trend as the "Fauci Effect." It's an interesting statistic because in response to the health crisis, students who may not have otherwise chosen to go to medical school decided to become doctors. Whatever the reason, it is admirable that so many young students were inspired to go to medical school, and I want to provide a resource to help the increasing number of aspiring physicians navigate the arduous, demanding, oftentimes punishing yet undoubtedly deeply fulfilling path to medicine. This is an honest account of my experiences in medical school. My hope is that by providing an outline of what the four years of medical school will look like, and more importantly through sharing my candid anecdotes and personal frustrations, readers will feel less alone when they face challenges along the way.

This book is for students embarking on the journey to become doctors. It is *also* for anyone who cares about someone who aspires to be a doctor. It is for the mothers, fathers, grandparents, partners, siblings, and dear friends of anyone on this path. I hope that in explaining what lies ahead it will foster an environment of inclusivity. We invite you into our life-long journey, and whole-heartedly welcome your support. It is powerful to feel *understood* by loved ones, and I hope this book brings understanding to those on the outside looking in.

I have been drawn to medicine well before I applied to medical school. My role models when shadowing doctors were those who were: tirelessly working out possible solutions, exceptionally empathetic, attentive to each patient, articulate and honest arbiters of knowledge while also supporting the vulnerable and sick. Working alongside these doctors has taught me how to be attentive to my patient's complex emotions and the circumstances that brought them to the hospital. I am learning what it feels like when your patient has a sense of impending doom about their death, and how quickly and unexpectedly death can come. I am learning how to apply clinical reasoning, putting pieces of a puzzle together to come to a diagnosis. I am learning to be patient, how to listen, when to speak, and when to allow for silence. I am also learning how to comfort those who are in physical pain and emotional distress.

I have reflected on the type of doctor that I want to become. My experiences as a student doctor have forced me to grapple with challenging questions: What happens when medicine is not enough? What happens when patients require more than medicine can offer? I want to be a doctor that runs toward these patients and not away, because I embrace our duty to be supportive until the end no matter the outcome.

Chapter II: On Advice

If I could give myself one piece of advice prior to starting medical school, it would be to *not let anything get in the way of being a compassionate person and doctor.*

Each person training to be a doctor has specific skills; traits that your mother or father may have identified in you at a young age or for which your friends call on you regularly. Don't lose those attributes. Instead, focus on amplifying them. Maybe you can be welcoming in an accessible way that is tremendously unique. Or you can focus on a project for 8 hours at a time without breaking focus. Maybe you're an empath; able to understand how someone is feeling without even asking. Medical school does not necessarily identify those unique individual unteachable skills.

Sometimes throughout medical school I have wondered why certain things are done that seem illogical. For example, in our first year of medical school, why did we spend over 10 hours every week in the anatomy lab dissecting a cadaver? I learned more about anatomy and human physiology from studying diagrams and working on cases in a group setting rather than hunched over a donor body silently separating large areas of fascia to complete the day's dissection. When other programs shortened the anatomy course, my medical school kept ours to nearly 12-weeks long—one of the longest Anatomy courses in the country. For over a week we dissected the different muscles of the feet, which seemed senseless to me. Due to significant pressure by students and an overwhelming shift throughout medical schools across the nation, the Anatomy course at my medical school was finally changed in the years immediately after my course. But I often wonder why it took so long, what was the reason behind the reluctance to change? In part, the school may have wanted to distinguish itself as having the most in-depth anatomy course in the country, perhaps hoping to impress prospective students. Regardless, this example shows that real change comes from within an institution. I feel empowered to have learned that thinking critically about a process and voicing concerns can result in positive changes for the next group of doctors.

The best skill I have learned from medical education is to remain true to myself. In this book I hope to discuss my journey through medical school in a transparent and open way. Ultimately, I can say without a doubt that I am grateful I have chosen this path. I look forward to my career as a doctor and I am happy I made the decision to become a physician. However, there have been many times in medical school where I felt powerless and alone. I want to discuss some of the emotional wounds that were inflicted in medical school. I hope that in discussing the challenges I faced, it might allow other medical students to feel less alone.

In my first year of medical school, we were evaluated while interviewing a patient. The patient interview is the conversation you have with your doctor usually starting with the question, "so what brings you in today?" Your job as the doctor is to figure out what is wrong, offer your sincere empathy, and do thorough detective work—making sure not to miss any key details.[2] After this mock interview, the 'patient' is asked to fill out an evaluation, and an observing physician also completes a thorough evaluation of your

---

[2] For example, a key detail might be that the patient began experiencing new symptoms of headache and nausea that coincided with beginning a new medication. This would raise suspicion for possible side-effects of the medication as the cause of the patient's symptoms (many drugs can cause headache and/or nausea).

skill as an interviewer. In my first 'objective structured clinical exam' (OSCE), as they are called at medical schools throughout the country, I received less than average marks on my interview from the physician evaluator. I was told my organization was off. It was not consistent with the handout given in class which followed a mnemonic for "remembering how to show empathy.[3]" I was also told that I didn't ask the patient about sexual history or recreational drug use (both of which seemed irrelevant to the case and felt like intrusive questions for me to ask at an initial appointment and could result in the patient closing off).

On the other hand, the patient, who I had just spent 30 minutes speaking with, evaluated me differently. She gave me high marks on my evaluation and wrote in the comments that

"In a short time upon meeting him, I felt I could share anything with the student doctor. He made me feel comfortable and listened to."

It felt really encouraging to read this review from the patient, I felt like my natural communication style resonated with the patient. It felt silly to abide by an acronym for empathy, but nevertheless I was advised by the doctor to adopt it to get a good score on future OSCE's.

---

[3] The acronym we learned was PEARLS which stands for partnership, empathy, apology, respect, legitimization, support. To me, it feels more natural to express this type of support organically in conversation with the patient, rather than, for example, offering an apology, "I'm sorry you are in pain" only after showing empathy "that sounds really painful." This approach seemed robotic and nonsensical to me. I had spent my life interacting with people and wondered why I would scrap my instincts to follow this new framework.

When I have been a patient myself, there have been instances where I have felt my doctor seemed emotionless and robotic. Through this experience with the OSCE early in medical school, I realized that the mechanical way in which some doctors communicate with patients could be a result of the type of advice I received from the observing physician during training. I am still navigating striking a balance between following convention and following my gut. Regarding interpersonal interaction with patients, I tend to communicate with patients the way I would want my doctor to speak with me or my parents. Instead of mining information from people I am caring for, inserting statements of empathy intermittently and using their story as a tool for reaching a diagnosis and treatment plan, I tend to view the patient as my partner—the Watson to my Sherlock, Robin to my Batman. Ultimately, I find this approach makes patients feel more comfortable, a part of the team, and *listened* to.

I had always assumed that the conventions of medicine were followed for a reason. Doctors have successfully cared for patients long before I entered the field and will continue to do so long after me. But I have come to learn that patients and doctors can both benefit from questioning some of the conventions. The patient presentation is a great example of this.[4] Roughly, the presentation follows the SOAP format, which is an acronym for subjective, objective, assessment, and plan

---

[4] The patient presentation is how doctors communicate about patients. In an academic hospital setting, the resident doctor will round (visit patients for whom the physician is responsible) on patients first thing in morning. The resident would then round on the patients again with the rest of the team and present the patients to the group in this conventional format.

(there is no shortage of acronyms in medicine). For example, the subjective portion, which is supposed to reflect the patient's *subjective* medical state might begin with a one-liner about the patient: *48-year-old female with a history of diabetes, depression, and alcohol use disorder presented to the hospital two days ago complaining of dry cough and shortness of breath.* Then typically it includes a description about the relevant positive and negative symptoms like: *The patient endorses a 'pounding' 8/10 headache located in the temples bilaterally that has been continuous for 4 days, has not improved with Tylenol, and is made worse with bright light. She is afebrile, denies nausea, vomiting, diarrhea.*

In the conventional SOAP format, the presentation would continue to include objective data: vital signs, physical examination, lab work, and imaging. Eventually, minutes later, the presentation includes the doctor's clinical assessment of the patient and their medical plan. I have never had two attending[5] doctors have the same expectations as to the exact format of the presentation. Despite the variability, most are passionate that the way they want the presentations is the correct and logical way. I have learned to ask on the first day working with a new attending what their

---

[5] Full-fledged physician, aka not a trainee anymore. The attending is essentially the boss of any medical team in the hospital. For example, if you found yourself in the unfortunate position of being a patient in the hospital, and in the even more unfortunate position of having a nice but visibly nervous 3rd year medical student on his first day of his surgery rotation struggling to remove a 'wound vac' from your leg (essentially a vacuum that is taped to a wound to prevent any fluid or infection from developing) you might say: "I need to speak with your attending physician!"

preferences are regarding the presentation. I have been told contradictory instructions about how presentations must be done. Some *expect* medical journal articles to be printed out and talked about to support the plan for each patient. Others want the fewest words possible to get through the entire thing.

Rounding on patients can be a lengthy process—I have rounded on a group of 8 patients that has taken over four hours because of the presentations. Most of the medical team have already read about the patient extensively in the chart, and the presentation is a redundant time-suck. It is true that presenting patients in this way might be more educational to the students on the team. But there must be another way to learn more efficiently that doesn't delay patient care and increase the length of hospital stays. While the medical team is on rounds, which often lasts from 7:30 am to 11:30 am, it takes the group's full attention. Now that we have the most current patient charts at our fingertips on our phones and computers (that are updated in real time), it is time to re-evaluate conventional patient presentations and rounding.

Individuals in the pursuit of becoming a doctor are subjected to a lot of unsolicited advice. For example, I have been told (by doctors) that if I can picture myself doing anything other than medicine, to do that. That being a doctor is now a more feasible career choice for women because it is not lucrative enough for men.[6] That most medical jobs will be *replaced* by artificial intelligence by the time I am finished with my training. That doctors don't receive the same respect from the public that they used to so it's not worth it anymore. Or my personal favorite: simply adding up the years of training it entails in my face (hint: it's a lot of years).

---

[6] I believe my response to this was "yikes." Simply too much to unpack here.

Once I was in medical school the advice kept coming. During my third year I was asked by a friend (who works in finance) what field I wanted to go into. When I responded that I was interested in Oncology, he replied "Oh, no. You'll get so burned out." I wasn't quite sure what this person meant or how he arrived at this conclusion, since he is not in the healthcare field. It almost seemed like the comment was second nature, perhaps he was simply regurgitating a line he had heard other people say. I wondered if outside of the field of medicine the term 'burn out' was becoming synonymous with 'doctor.'

So, I did some research and discovered that physician burnout starts early. 44% of *medical students* report burn out. This is a time when most medical trainees are in their mid-20's and are only just *starting* to see patients. Interestingly, compassion is inversely related to burnout, which is an encouraging finding because it shows that job satisfaction and happiness can be within an individual's control.[7] Expressing compassion, caring for others, may not only be helpful to the society at large but also serves the medical professional. The more focus shifts away from self-interest, considering patient's needs intently ultimately can combat burnout. Average suicide rates in medicine are double what they are in other professions.[8] Although it is important to acknowledge burnout, simply tossing out the term loosely does not do it justice. It is a psychological syndrome that can be explained by a response to

---

[7] Trzeciak, S., Mazzarelli, A., Compassionomics: *The Revolutionary Scientific Evidence that Caring Makes a Difference.* May 10, 2019.
[8] Dutheil, Frédéric et al. "Suicide among physicians and health-care workers: A systematic review and meta-analysis." *PloS one* vol. 14,12 e0226361. 12 Dec. 2019, doi:10.1371/journal.pone.0226361

chronic stressors. It can manifest in many ways including: loss of motivation, feeling trapped or defeated, detached, cynical, decreased satisfaction, and fatigue. Remaining true to yourself and connecting to the reasons you pursued medicine in the first place, identifying your *uniqueness*, may serve as one antidote to the frustrations within the medical field.

This book is not an attempt to solve the enumerable problems with medical education that occur starting with pre-medical courses in undergraduate school through medical school, residency, and fellowship. I plan on identifying many of these issues and offering my thoughts on how these problems can be dealt with on an individual level no matter how frustrating or unjust. Because whether these problems are fixed before your medical training, you will always face unnecessary challenges that are out of your control. Developing tools to deal with these unnecessary challenges is important because we need good, rational people to become doctors, and withstanding a nonsensical, never-ending, and oftentimes broken process does not select for individuals who necessarily value logic. Being prepared to learn from difficult systems and persevere, is a skill that can bring you clarity, strength, and peace.

Chapter III: The preclinical years

Medical school is 4 years. Traditionally, the first two years have been in the classroom, taking what are called "pre-clinical" courses.[9] The following two years are in the hospital, working with patients full-time. Over the last 5-10 years there has been a general shift in medical education to shorten the "pre-clinical" years—some programs limiting them to 15-18 months of straight classes, followed by hospital-based training. This shift allows students to have more time experiencing patient-centered training during medical school and allows them to explore more elective rotations.[10]

The pre-clinical courses include histology, which pertains to studying normal and diseased tissues under a microscope, and anatomy, which involves studying the

---

[9] 'Clinical' means patient focused. Clinical studies might include studying the treatment regimen for a patient with heart failure. 'Pre-clinical' studies would pertain to studying the science behind heart failure; like how the cardiac muscle cells lose their ability to stretch over time. The science behind disease is *pathophysiology*. These terms are also often used in the context of research. Clinical research, for example, means research that pertains directly to patient care. This contrasts with 'basic science' research—which would be research you might expect from a 'wet-lab,' (i.e., lab coats, standing at a lab bench, chemicals, hard-core science). Somewhere in between clinical and basic science research is *translational* research. Meaning, research that is directly *translatable* to the patient bedside.

[10] An elective rotation may be in a specific subspecialty a student is interested in that is not part of the core curriculum such as gastroenterology or cardiothoracic surgery.

form and function of the human body and historically includes human cadaver dissection. During this time students study diseases and how they work, how they are treated, and what causes them. For example, we study biochemistry, pharmacology, and immunology.

Anatomy lab

Beginning the anatomy course in the first year of medical school, it seemed like we were embarking on a rite of passage. The course started with a ceremony in honor of the cadaver donations. My anatomy group, 'met' our cadaver for the first time and respectfully acknowledged the life and death of what some call our 'first patient.'

I felt like it was a respectful way to begin the anatomy course. It allowed us to think about the life of the cadaver and express gratitude for the donation. I imagine that one reason why people decide to donate their body to medical schools is because they want to help to educate the future generation of doctors. I have also learned in speaking with geriatric social workers that many people choose to donate their body to avoid the high cost of a burial—they do not wish to financially burden their family members. Donating to medical schools is free.

Some of the dissections were beautiful and fascinating. Particularly, I was awestruck when we successfully removed the heart and examined all its different chambers. I was amazed by how large and muscular it felt in my hand. The same is true for when we removed the liver—it felt huge to me, and it was shaped strikingly like its depictions in textbooks. It looked cartoonish. I will never forget which side of the body it is on after that dissection, since we were standing over the body for hours cutting the correct branches of the hepatic veins to keep the organ in one piece.

I soon realized that the anatomy lab is not for the faint of heart. To be honest, I did not enjoy the dissections— I prepared for each day in the lab, reading the instructions for the dissection that we would have to do the next day, and sometimes they horrified me. Particularly horrifying was the unit on the head and neck.

During the head dissection, my anatomy group was tasked with executing a 'hemi-section' which is cutting through the cadaver's head longitudinally, splitting it down the middle from the apex of the head, through the cranium and neck to the top of the larynx. Spending hours doing dissections like this I often wondered: what is the benefit of this? I kept reassuring myself that it was to gain a better understanding of the anatomy of the region.

This procedure was traumatizing for me. My role in the group was typically not as hands-on as some of the other students. I helped explain what area to dissect, where to stop cutting, and helped prop up various parts of the cadaver to assist in the dissections. A couple of aspiring surgeons in my group enjoyed performing most of the actual dissections—and I was happy to let them. On this day, however, we used a bone saw and a table saw to perform the gruesome dissection. I performed the hemisecting of the head and neck since I had the most experience with these tools and was physically the largest in the group (cutting thick bone and tissue with a blunt table-saw requires a bit of elbow grease).

It took me about thirty minutes. The rest of my group silently watched as I cut through skin, fascia, cartilage, bone, and brain. The sound of manually cutting the skull of the cadaver is seared in my memory. Afterward, dripping in sweat and feeling a bit nauseous,

I felt guilty about what I had done. Over the couple of months prior to this dissection, I had grown connected with the cadaver, and this was the first procedure that rendered it unrecognizable. It looked like something you might see in a horror movie. In the anatomy lab, most of my peers carried themselves confidently and appeared to have no problem with the dissections. I left that day in the lab feeling frazzled and alone. At the end of that dissection, examining the anatomy of the region on the cadaver, I couldn't help but feel like I learned it better on the computer simulations and pictures from the textbook. I didn't feel like there was any point to what I had done, which is what still leaves me disturbed today.

Concurrent with the Anatomy course and continuing after its completion, we study the *physiology* of each organ system, which is how an organ system (e.g., the circulatory system) works when it is functioning normally (i.e., not diseased). Then we study all the things that can go wrong in that organ system. For example, in our cardiovascular disease course we first studied how the heart beats, the electrical signals that pulsate through individual cardiac muscle cells called *myocytes*. We learned about the fluid dynamics in the cardiovascular system: how much blood pumps with each beat, where the blood is distributed throughout the body, the different types of vessels that bring blood to and from the heart, and the different ways to image and visualize the heart. After several weeks of learning this physiology, we transition to learning about the different diseases that affect the heart. For example, students learn about the difference between dilated cardiomyopathy and restrictive cardiomyopathy, heart failure, and myocardial infarctions. This process is repeated in studying the other organ systems in the human body like the lungs, kidneys, endocrine system, neurology, psychiatry, etc...

Throughout this first phase of medical school, medical students are also learning about clinical medicine and practicing skills interacting with patients. First- and second-year students are likely in a course that meets once or twice a week to practice gathering information from patients (a process called the 'patient interview' or 'taking a history' from a patient). At this point, medical students are learning how to perform a proper physical examination (i.e., listening to the heart and lungs etc.) and are starting to see patients of their own in the hospital under the supervision of a physician-educator.

Chapter IV: How to Study in Medical School

Doctors should be good at learning and retaining new information. Patients expect doctors to have a large fund of knowledge and defer to their expertise based on years of training and experience. However, some of what doctors learn in medical school turns out to be wrong. The way the scientific community thought about bacteria, for example, has greatly evolved over the last few decades. The medical community has learned to understand that all bacteria are not the enemy but can serve as a crucial part of immune health, nutrition, and digestion. Still, building a foundation of knowledge is an important first step in the path to becoming a doctor and our ability to continue learning even after training will serve us well in modifying the fund of knowledge acquired in medical school. We can then ask questions, engage in scientific research to advance the field of medicine, and contribute to our evolving understanding of human health. People say that medical school is like drinking from a firehose. There is a tremendous amount to learn in a short period of time and so we must adapt our way of learning to accommodate it. Learning in medical school should be as simple as possible. When you learn simply, your methods can be applied broadly. Throughout my many years of studying, I identified that for me, there are three main components to learning: acquisition, repetition, and testing.

Acquisition
Knowledge acquisition is how you acquire new information. For example, this can be from formal lectures at your medical school, from textbooks, videos on the topic, or even directly from answer explanations in question banks. Before a course begins in the preclinical years, pick one or two resources for a class

or field of study. And that may change from one course to the next. Resources will often change as the years go by, but you should always ask your colleagues what resources they are using, and you should not ask professors or attendings what resources they might recommend because in my experience they are often outdated or redundant. The best study tips always come from the person who just finished what you are about to start. For example, prior to beginning our course on the endocrine system, I learned that our professor was extremely thorough and engaging. Endocrinology pertains to hormones in the body, organs that secrete hormones or respond to them. It covers many different organ systems and diseases. So, I decided to utilize the course lectures as my primary resource for knowledge acquisition. This was uncommon for me in medical school. I found my endocrinology professor to be exceptional—he was engaging, made me laugh out loud during lecture, his lecture slides were organized, and he covered all the most important topics carefully. Ideally, this would be the case for every subject, especially because we are paying so much for tuition. But since we all have different learning styles and preferences, the one-size-fits-all approach to learning that has been the tradition for so long does not make sense now that there are an infinite number of resources at our fingertips. Giving students the freedom to engage with material in the way that best suits them is important. Allowing students to learn new concepts in an individualized way was one of the many areas where my medical school excelled. Learning how to learn is one of the most important aspects of higher education. My knowledge acquisition process for the Cardiology course was much different than Endocrinology. One of the most popular online learning resources for medical students is called Boards and Beyond, which contains many short video lectures from Dr. Jason Ryan.[11] He is

---

[11] https://boardsbeyond.com/homepage

a Cardiologist, and his videos on the subject were particularly strong. So, I used all his videos on Cardiology as my primary source. I ignored the medical school lectures altogether. There are many complex categories of drugs within the subject of Cardiology, so I added one more online resource called Sketchy Medical, which is a visual learning platform that utilizes narrative arcs, mnemonics, and drawing that I found particularly helpful for learning drugs.[12] As you can tell, my approach to knowledge acquisition in my Endocrine course was much different than my Cardiology course. I did it this way because I discovered those resources were strongest on the topic. I did not think the Endocrinology videos were very good on Boards and Beyond, and I did not think my medical school lectures were helpful to me for learning Cardiology. Being flexible in this way also helped keep me engaged and excited for new approaches each course. There were times I committed to a resource based on a recommendation from a peer but had to change a couple weeks into the course because it wasn't best for me. This process is effective because over time you get to know yourself more deeply: as a learner and thinker.

Repetition
Carefully make thoughtful notecards on a virtual platform like anki or quizlet.[13,14] Make notecards instead of 'taking notes.' For Cardiology for example, the front of the card might be a question or a fill in the blank. On the back of the card is the answer along with further notes on the topic to remind yourself the context or an image that you found useful on the topic. Notecards assess for discrete testable facts. An entire

---

[12] https://www.sketchy.com/
[13] https://apps.ankiweb.net/
[14] https://quizlet.com/

concept can be boiled down to one or two short questions that can be on the front of a notecard.

Notecards are more useful when virtual and can include screenshots of helpful images or background information for context. Eventually they should include screenshots of questions about the topic. You will encounter a practice question on a topic that covers information in your notecard or relating to it. That is when you add it to your card. Fewer is always better. It's better to know you will do 20 notecards a day then to over-extend and create too many notecards. You might do 200 notecards a day for a few days, but you will fall behind and then end up doing zero.

You might put an image of a pressure-volume loop tracing on the front of the card and ask: how would you describe the cardiac condition in this patient? On the back of the card, you might write the answer 'dilated cardiomyopathy.' Then you might have images of a normal pressure-volume loop tracing, compared to dilated cardiomyopathy, restricted cardiomyopathy, etc. Then you might write in some of the causes of those conditions you have trouble remembering, or you might put in a practice question that shows tricky pressure-volume loops, or the link to a video you thought was useful describing how patients compensate for reduced stroke volume. Many notecard platforms allow for spaced repetition. Meaning, you can decide in how many days you want to repeat a card based on how well you think you know it. If you don't know the content of the card well, you would want to see it again tomorrow. If you feel comfortable with a card, you might not want to see it again for a month. If you make cards carefully and review them mindfully, then you can maintain your card repetition even after you finish a course in medical school. All your hard work studying will not be lost, and you can retain information long-term.

Testing

Pay for access to question banks or ask your medical school to pay for subscriptions for your entire class. I like Uworld and Amboss most for questions.[15,16] The explanation for the correct answer, and explanations about why the distractors are wrong is truly phenomenal. Once you have reached a critical point acquiring information and practicing repetitious learning with your notecards, you are ready to start having fun with practice questions. Eventually doing a set of practice questions will feel cozy and familiar. Like a fish slipping into water. Do quality questions slowly, learn to let go of details you think are not important. Learn concepts well the first time. If you are stumped or frustrated, take a deep breath and a break and come back to it. Do not overdo it. Do not let stress or anxiety guide your study plan. Determine what you intend to cover before you sit down and do not do more questions than that mindlessly. As an exam approaches, do practice questions under time constrictions. Your attention span will increase with practice. My approach to questions in an exam setting is common. Read the last line of the question stem, skim the answer choices, read the entire question stem, identify abnormal lab results, eliminate incorrect answer choices, and finally select an answer. This method should be practiced too.

---

[15] https://www.uworld.com/
[16] https://www.amboss.com/us

Chapter V: Beyond the pre-clinical years

Once medical students are done with the 'lecture years' they start what was traditionally called "clerkships," which most people now call '3rd year rotations.' This year you rotate through all the same disciplines as your classmates. The duration of each rotation typically lasts somewhere between 5-8 weeks depending on the school. The rotations are quite general, spanning a broad swath of practice settings and clinical exposure.[17] Historically this year is the time students are thinking about which specialty they might want to pursue, sampling the broad categories of medicine to decide which type of residency program to apply to. For example, perhaps a student is considering pursuing internal medicine as a career, but unexpectedly feels greatly fulfilled by the work on the psychiatry rotation. Perhaps they have a great preceptor[18] for the psychiatry rotation—one who inspires them to pursue the field. This is one of the reasons why the 3rd year of medical

---

[17] For example, at my school our 3rd-year rotations included: internal medicine, general surgery, obstetrics and gynecology, pediatrics, psychiatry, neurology, radiology, and family medicine. Students could be rotating at a small practice in an urban setting or in a suburban area. Students might rotate at various large academic centers that are affiliated with the medical school. Sometimes students are placed based on ranking preferences, other times it is a random allocation.

[18] Preceptor is the attending doctor who oversees the medical student, who the medical student reports to and who grades the medical student. Oftentimes the preceptor is an attending physician who has an interest in teaching, other times attendings are simply required to precept as part of their contract with the hospital.

school carries so much weight. Deciding which field of medicine to commit yourself to for an entire career is a daunting decision. This is also made tougher since the rotations are relatively short—you may not get a ton of personal experience in each of the specialties before it's time to decide.

Nowadays, it is common to decide what residency to apply to before even beginning the 3rd year, since it is becoming more common to have some research experience in the field prior to applying to residency.[19] According to the NRMP residency match data from 2020, the governing body that conducts residency match,[20] matched applicants in internal medicine have an average of 6.2 abstracts, presentations, and publications prior to residency applications in their 4th

---

[19] *National Resident Matching Program: Charting Outcomes in the Match.* (2020). NRMP.Org. https://mk0nrmp3oyqui6wqfm.kinstacdn.com/wp-content/uploads/2020/07/Charting-Outcomes-in-the-Match-2020_MD-Senior final.pdf

[20] The residency match is the process by which graduating medical students land their first job after medical school. It is a one-of-a-kind job placement process. In the final year of medical school, applicants apply to residency programs in the specialty of their choosing and embark on the next step in their training called 'residency.' To attain a position at a program, applicants must officially submit their *ranked* list of preferred programs where they interviewed, and the programs *rank* all the applicants they interviewed in order of preference. The process is called residency 'match' because an algorithm then 'matches' candidates to their respective training programs. The results of the match are *binding* and are revealed on the same day nationwide in March every year. If this career-defining ritual seems barbaric to you, that's because it is.

year of medical school. A significant amount of time and work is required to complete research projects, and so starting research later in medical school makes it difficult to be involved in over 6 projects prior to residency applications. This is compared to matched applicants in internal medicine completing a mean of 4.4 abstracts, presentations, and publications in NRMP's 2016 survey results. This number continues to grow as programs become more competitive over time, in large part due to applicants' desire to do more because they want to bulk up their CV. Anecdotally, this tendency to raise the bar is rampant in the path to becoming a doctor. The culture of one-upmanship is not specific to medicine, but with so much time dedicated to the specific career path, anxiety can weigh heavily and doing as much as possible to avoid restlessness can be a temporary relief from anxiety. Why only do four research projects when you can cram in an additional two projects during a research year? The attitude is that more publications is better, regardless of the quality of the research or whether the student is passionate about the work. The old saying in academia suggesting "publish or perish," has permeated into the minds of eager anxiety-ridden medical students. Only 'perishing' in this case is not getting fired or failing to become a tenured professor, rather it's failing to match into a top choice residency.

The fourth and final year of medical school is characterized by *applying* to residency. Most applications are submitted in September of fourth year, interviews are held throughout the winter and students find out where they match in March.

Chapter VI: USMLE Step 1 and 2

Medical students typically have a major exam every 2 weeks throughout the preclinical years of medical school. In the past 5-10 years, most medical schools have shifted to a pass/fail system for the preclinical years. This helped combat the unnecessary competitiveness that plagues medical students (and may be the reason for their successful admission to medical school in the first place). These exams are written and distributed by the school for each of their courses. But since there are usually no letter grades for these courses, there is another quantitative way to differentiate students when applying for residency programs. This is where the United States Medical Licensing Examination (USMLE) comes into play.[21]

The USMLE is a three-step examination for medical licensure in the U.S. It has been around for a long time; it was first distributed in 1922.[22] The goal of these exams is to "assess a physician's ability to apply knowledge, concepts, and principles, and to demonstrate fundamental patient-centered skills that are important in health and disease and that constitute the basis of safe and effective patient care."[23] Medical students take Step 1 and Step 2 exams in medical school. Traditionally, Step 1 is taken after preclinical years are completed and before students start the clerkship year. Step 2 is taken after the clerkship year

[21] The USMLE is owned by two entities, the Federation of State Medical Boards (FSM) and the National Board of Medical Examiners (NBME)

[22] Kies, Susan, and Mary Shultz. "Proposed changes to the United States Medical Licensing Examination: impact on curricula and libraries." *Journal of the Medical Library Association: JMLA* vol. 98,1 (2010): 12-6. doi:10.3163/1536-5050.98.1.007

[23] https://www.usmle.org/

around the time students are applying for residency. These tests are 8 and 9 hours long respectively, taken at Prometric test centers, and had both always been scored numerically until 2022, when the USMLE announced Step 1 will change to pass/fail grading.

Up until this change, Step 1 had been one of the most important factors a residency program used to consider whether to interview an applicant.[24] Competitive specialties like neurosurgery, ENT, plastic surgery, and dermatology have cut-off scores, below which they will not consider an applicant (cut-offs that are well above the national average). During my time as a medical student, just before the shift to pass fail was made, step 1 anxiety seemed astronomically high. Some of my peers began studying for the exam on the first day of medical school. Students often skipped lectures so they could spend more time studying for Step 1. However, in their explanation for the grading change, the USMLE concedes that the licensing exam was never designed to precisely differentiate intellect with a high degree of specificity. This begs the question: Why did it take decades to change an imperfect grading system that had such a profound impact on selecting applications? Even though the governing body that develops the USMLE exams, the National Board of Medical Examiners (NBME), is a non-profit organization that has been tax-exempt since 1937, the revenue from NBME's programs,[25] nearly quadrupled from 2001 ($47.5 million) to 2019 (180.7 million).[26]

---

[24] Mun, Frederick et al. "Internal medicine residency program director perceptions of USMLE Step 1 pass/fail scoring: A cross-sectional survey." *Medicine* vol. 100,15 (2021): e25284. doi:10.1097/MD.0000000000025284
[25] The NBME (National Board of Medical Examiners) is a non-profit which develops and manages assessments of health care professionals. It develops the

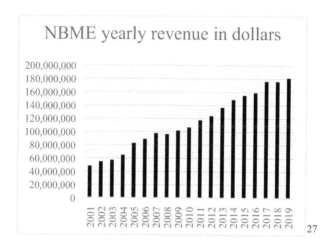

NBME yearly revenue in dollars

One might wonder why students were expected to pay over $600 just to sit for each exam (not to mention hundreds more on test-prep materials) if the exam, by its own admission, is so lacking in key statistical measures like specificity? Even though there is a high degree of variability and imprecision in the scoring process, the difference between a 235 and a 245 on the exam for example, could very well mean the difference between a student matching into their dream specialty of orthopedic surgery and not even being considered for a position because they did not meet the 240-score threshold. In other words, the exam was being used as a

USMLE in partnership with the Federation of State Medical Boards.
[26] "National Board of Medical Examiners (NBME)." National Board of Medical Examiners (NBME) | Philadelphia, PA | Cause IQ, https://www.causeiq.com/organizations/national-board-of-medical-examiners,231352238/.
[27] Ken Schwencke, Mike Tigas. "National Board of Medical Examiners - Nonprofit Explorer." ProPublica, 9 May 2013, https://projects.propublica.org/nonprofits/organizations/231352238.

tool to weed-out applicants even though it was designed as a competency exam—a threshold that students needed to clear before advancing to the next step in training.

Instead of focusing on the medical school coursework, students study using test prep materials. As the importance of the exam increased, so did the quality (and cost) of test prep materials, and the average score steadily skyrocketed from 221 in 2008 to 232 in 2019.[28]

Obviously, residency programs found it useful to rely on a quantitative exam, using the numerical score to determine if an applicant would be interviewed. Perhaps the exam was useful to residency programs as a simple and quick way to decrease the size of the pool of applicants it was considering. This would make the review process more economical—they wouldn't have to hire as many people to review applications. Maybe they wanted to only select the highest scoring applicants because they viewed it as an accurate predictor of future performance on board exams. If the residents were better test takers, maybe they would not have to study as much for the board exams during residency (Step 3), which means they could work harder in the hospital and focus on patient care.

Two parties are at fault, which led to a vicious cycle. Residency programs, inundated with more applications than it could read, and ill-equipped to carefully read them all—relied heavily on the exam's quantitative result to weed out applicants and make their job less time-consuming. As applicants realized this, demand increased for exam-specific educational resources for

---

[28] USMLE Score Interpretation Guidelines. https://www.usmle.org/sites/default/files/2021-08/USMLE_Step_Examination_Score_Interpretation_Guidelines.pdf.

students to attain better scores. The NBME was complicit regarding residency programs misusing and over-emphasizing its exam results (based on an imprecise, inequitable exam) and continued raising the stakes for its own financial gain.

Whatever the reason for residency program's increasing reliance on Step 1 scores to select its resident doctors, and despite the NBME's clear financial incentives, they finally made a drastic change in the grading of the test. Instead of redesigning the exam or offering a new solution to replace the clear reliance on these exams by residency programs, as of January 2022, Step 1 changed to pass/fail.

There are benefits and challenges to this change. Residency programs must figure out another way to weed out students and may look for some other quantitative measure to compare students from different medical schools. For international medical graduates applying for a residency program in the US, attaining a high score on step 1 was a way to catch the attention of residency program directors. Additionally, scoring high on the exam was a way for students from less prestigious medical schools to distinguish themselves. But scoring in the top quartile on the exam is not necessarily an indication of intelligence. Like many standardized exams, a high score on the exam is more easily attainable if you have the luxury of time, resources, and money.[29] Test prep and question banks are expensive. There are enough companies selling test prep materials for these exams that a medical student

---

[29] Carmody, Bryan. "A Non-MBA's Guide to NBME Revenue in 9 Simple Charts." The Sheriff of Sodium, 24 May 2020, https://thesheriffofsodium.com/2019/02/01/a-non-mbas-guide-to-nbme-revenue-in-9-simple-charts/.

who wants to cover their bases could easily rack up a thousand-dollar bill to pay for the materials.

Many predict that the focus will shift from step 1 to step 2. The step 2 examination historically has been less important for residency applications. But now, as the only remaining numerical value on a student's application, students are shifting their focus to the second USMLE exam.[30]

Medical schools generally do not vary significantly in their curriculum or design. Most nowadays have an initial preclinical portion which varies in duration as I have described. Some schools have a more traditional two full school years with a summer break in between. Most programs have shifted to going straight through for a period of 11-15 months. Some programs still have letter grades for this period, but most have shifted to a pass-fail system. Regardless of the design, all medical students start medical school with a rigorous period of learning, studying, and testing; and testing continues throughout medical school and beyond.

Admittedly, I personally scored above the national average for matched US MD applicants on both Step 1 and Step 2, which was a significant asset on my residency application. But my score is attributed to my privileged position that I was able to purchase the top question banks and study tools. Had I not studied using those expensive resources, I would not have done as

---

[30] Being a good test taker is the most important factor in doing well in medical school. Whether or not being a good test taker makes you a better doctor is up for debate. But what is not up for debate is that if you are not a good test taker medical schools and residencies may view you as a liability. Residency programs want residents who pass certification exams with ease so that they can be of more value to the hospital.

well. In many ways the score on this exam has become a surrogate marker for performance in medical school. But it's important to understand the questionable validity of the claim that scoring well on these exams correlates with better clinical performance in residency and beyond. It's important to question whether the test is fair, useful, and if it achieves its intended purpose.

Chapter VII: Narrowing in on the Clinical Years

After learning in the classroom, the next period of medical school is the clinical years, where students are expected to both work in the hospital learning on rotations and study intensely outside of work. This is an incredibly exciting time for medical students because for the first time, you will be in the hospital every day and will be responsible for patients. You'll report to your team and work closely with attending physicians and residents. Medical students are thrilled to be seeing patients. This is what we have worked so hard for many years to do.

Most programs use a grading system for clinical rotations. For example, at my medical school, attendings and residents that worked with medical students would be sent a formal evaluation afterward.

The categories might span "physical examination" to "professionalism" including pretty much most categories you can think of to evaluate a person (even "integrity" as a category). This way of evaluating is quite subjective. What one evaluator marks a 5/5, another might mark a 3/5. On top of this, evaluators might have worked with you for a day or an afternoon, and yet their evaluation of you will count just as much as someone who works with you for 2 weeks. Furthermore, while a score of 3/5 is perfectly 'adequate' for all the questions on the evaluation, if a student averaged this score across all evaluators it would result in a failing grade of 60% (they would have to repeat the clerkship). Essentially, simply meeting adequate competency levels is not enough. A score of 3/5 regarding clinical judgement on the scoring rubric indicates: "[Student] prioritizes patient information and generates [an] adequate, basic differential diagnosis" is quite literally not good enough to pass the clerkship. This misleading grading system is often not communicated appropriately to all the physicians (who are incredibly busy) that a student works with and who must fill out these evaluations. Because of this, 3rd year is characterized by hyper-vigilant medical students, terrified of rubbing anyone the wrong way out of fear that someone will give them a bad evaluation. This way of grading encourages falsehood since realistically, someone who briefly supervises you likely is not able to accurately evaluate for these traits.[31]

One of my friends named Ben told me that he was given a 2/5 in the category of "integrity" on one of the evaluations. This evaluator spent one afternoon with Ben. I joked that maybe the physician saw him find a 20-dollar-bill in the parking lot and instead of turning it into the security desk, he pocketed it. Ben assured me that nothing happened out of the ordinary that afternoon. When Ben asked the physician about the evaluation, he stated "2/5 is good!"

At the end of each rotation, there is a standardized nationwide exam that is administered by the NBME. 110 questions that students answer in 2:45 minutes on the last day of the rotation. The score on this exam will count towards the overall clerkship grade to varying degrees. Typically, somewhere in the 20-40% of your overall grade. These exams are difficult, and

---

[31] Once I was reduced to a question mark. An evaluator once wrote about me "As a valued member of the team, ? consistently demonstrated a deep fund of knowledge…" This pretty much summed up my sense of anonymity as a third-year medical student. The fact that some evaluators simplified their evaluations to plugging in names into pre-formed sentences, made me realize the system was an epic failure.

performance is often tough to predict and, in my case, varied greatly.

For example, my first rotation as a third-year medical student was Psychiatry/Neurology. The rotation was 6-weeks long, and I decided to start studying for the exam my first week—this seemed like an early start based on my friends' study schedules, but I wanted to be as prepared as possible for my first shelf exam because I didn't know what to expect. I have found that I learn best from doing practice questions, so I purchased two different question banks—each one had roughly 400 questions. If I wanted to complete them all, I calculated that over the 42 days of the rotation, I had to do 20 questions a day. This was no easy feat, because sometimes a question would introduce a new topic I needed to learn. Sometimes 20 questions could take 3-4 hours to review, especially when starting a new clerkship. The questions have elaborate explanations, and so I would study the explanations and make notecards on the information I learned. Every day I did 20 questions and reviewed my notecards. By the end of the rotation, I knew roughly 1,000 notecards cold, based on the high-yield questions. I could sense that I was learning a lot based on topics that came up in the hospital during the rotation. I knew the answers to questions the psychiatrists asked me, and I knew the various drug classes for my patients and could recommend a treatment plan based on my newly developed knowledge.

I was vigilant—I felt that I could not miss a day studying or else I would fall behind in my schedule.[32] Studying had to get done in the early morning hours before I got to the hospital, and in the late evenings after I got home. In my last week of the rotation, I

---

[32] This was the method I used for studying for all my rotations moving forward.

purchased the practice exams that are released by the
NBME—there were 3 of them for this exam. I
remember thinking that the questions on the practice
exams were difficult, and the question stems were
lengthy—I was pressed for time to get through them all
before the end of the exam. I was scoring in the high
70s, my best score was 81%. This was disheartening
because based on data from the previous years, the
average score on this shelf exam at my medical school
was an 88%. In general, if I was scoring close to the
average for my medical school, I knew I was in great
shape. My medical school is full of extremely smart
and stellar test takers (and people).

I studied hard every day for 40 days; I could articulate
the subtle differences between personality disorders and
recalled all the different mechanisms of psychiatric
drugs and their side-effect profiles, but I was scoring
lower than the average on the practice exams.
Regardless, I remained optimistic and convinced myself
that I could outperform my scores on the practice
exams. I resolved to simply do my best on the exam, to
not let exam nerves get in the way, and to stay focused,
moving quickly through the questions instead of
allowing myself to waste time if I got stumped by a
particular question.[33] I had developed a clear approach

---

[33] Through High School, College, and my pre-med
postbacc program I struggled with test anxiety. I often
couldn't sleep the night before an exam and struggled
with stomach distress the morning of exams. I had
taken the white-knuckle approach throughout this time.
I simply gritted my teeth and pushed through it. I was
lucky to never have any serious meltdowns during
exams, but it always seemed like a possibility. I would
push through the anxiety, take the exam, and forget
how taxing the exam-taking process was for me until
the next one. I assumed others dealt with the same
thing. Once I got to medical school and exams were so

through medical school for both studying and exam-taking. Part of that approach was dedicating myself to stillness and a calm mindset during exams. This was sometimes easier said than done.

In my psychiatry shelf exam, I was shocked by how few questions I was sure of. I felt I could narrow the answer choices to 2 or 3 options, but then would have to guess the answer. The question stems were even longer and more convoluted than the practice exams. There was a ton of information given in the question about a patient that did not ultimately have much to do with the diagnosis or answer choices. The patients in the questions showed a combination of symptoms I had not seen before. By the time I was halfway through the exam, I realized I only had an hour left. I had taken well over half the time to answer the questions so far and was not even confident I had answered many of them correctly. My heart sank and I began to panic. I thought to myself, "I'm going to have to re-take this exam. Even after all my studying. You blew it, Adam."

I had roughly 50 minutes to complete 55 questions. I decided to change my approach, I told myself—I'm just

frequent (roughly every 1-2 weeks), I had the maturity to reflect on my relationship with exams. The full-immersion method helped. I didn't have time to work myself up leading up to exams. They simply came and went, and it was on to the next one. I became desensitized to exams and even grew to enjoy them once I was able to quiet my mind and focus on problem solving. I never thought that eventually I would be able to eagerly walk into very consequential exams, like Step 1 and Step 2, with a slow heartbeat, clear mind, and dry palms. I am proud of this, and grateful medical school gave me the opportunity to confront fear in this way. Ultimately, perhaps that is the most important reason to take exams in the first place.

going to read the answer choices and skim the question to get the pertinent information, decide on the answer and go to the next one. My friend Ben and I later nicknamed this the, "wild, wild, west" approach to test-taking. We were cowboys out there—facing unpredictable terrain and unfriendly territory. I flew through the rest of the exam, not even reading most of the question prompts. I was frustrated that I put myself in this position. Timing usually was not an issue for me on exams throughout my life up until this point. I answered the last 10-15 questions of the exam in 3 minutes. I left feeling awful. I wasn't sure if I passed the exam.

I had the following week off before my next rotation and so my wife and our dog escaped to the Hudson Valley for the week. During that time, I was fixated on my score. I refreshed the page on my phone all day to check if my score was released.

A few days in I checked my score and was pleasantly surprised to see a score of 93%. At first, I was relieved. I had outperformed the average by 5 percentage points. Then, I felt disappointed in myself that I let the exam results trickle into my mind and take over. It had ruined the first couple days of my vacation.

I wondered; how did this even happen? The practice exams weren't even within 10 points of my score. These practice exams were comprised of questions that had been retired from old shelf exams—I assumed the practice tests might be designed to *underpredict* actual performance. This was giving the NBME practice exams too much credit. In subsequent shelf exams, the NBME practice exams *over*-predicted my score.[34]

---

[34] Most drastically on my OBGYN rotation, when I averaged a 94% on the 3 NBME practice shelf exams and ended with an 80% on the real thing.

Walking into the shelf exams I never knew what to expect. Taking the exams felt like a bloodbath and walking out of the exams I never felt like I did well or demonstrated my knowledge appropriately. It seemed like my Surgery shelf exam was filled with medicine questions, a rotation I wouldn't do for months. On my Pediatrics shelf exam there was a lot of psychiatry—I was lucky I had already done that rotation. Despite the long hours of meticulous studying, I felt like there was no guarantee that I even passed the exam. Things I learned in the hospital taking care of patients did not appear on exams. Over 90% of the material tested on shelf exams I had to learn from studying outside of the hospital. There is a tremendous amount to learn for the first time on each rotation and taking care of patients in the hospital simply didn't cover it all. For example, an entire week of my general surgery rotation was in bariatric surgery—such a narrow view of surgery that would not be tested at all.

This realization made it so that my fellow third-year medical students and I viewed the hospital work as a chore rather than a learning opportunity. Being in the hospital became a distraction from our *learning* to prepare for the exam. Instead of focusing on improving our communication skills on our teams in the hospital, and spending time with our patients, I felt the pull of my question banks and the notecards I had to memorize. I am not alone in this. I once saw a fellow medical student doing notecards on his phone *while* speaking with a patient. Students took their sick days to study leading up to the shelf exams. There simply wasn't enough time in the day to learn. On my surgery rotation, when we were required to work in the hospital from 6:00 am to 7:00 pm, I would often wake-up at 3:00 am to study beforehand because I knew I'd be too exhausted at the end of the day.

These types of exams would have been my worst nightmare before medical school. The unpredictability coupled with the importance and permanence of the result might have sent me spiraling. But ultimately when I was faced with this difficult challenge, I called on tools that I had developed to keep anxiety in check and prevent the exam from taking up too much space in my life. I forced myself to emphasize the *learning* rather than the testing. I told myself that the score on the exam does not reflect my self-worth. Rather, the process of learning and completing the rotation with the knowledge that I gave my best effort *to all aspects* of the rotation[35] is what I should be proud of. I considered, "what's the worst that can happen?" And this made the possibility of underperforming or even failing the exam seem less consequential.

Leading up to my third-year surgery rotation, I was eager to get into the OR. I wanted to scrub into surgeries and work with my hands. I was not necessarily interested in pursuing surgery as a career choice, but I had not ruled it out. I chose to rotate at the main hospital associated with my medical school so that I could brush shoulders with the best. I literally looked up to surgeons on billboards over the interstate highway as I drove throughout the region, which touted the surgical prowess of my hospital system. It was an exciting time to learn from these heroic role models. I was eager to meet the surgeons and study their behavior.

Many of the surgeons lived up to my high expectations. On the ENT service, I recall one surgeon who carefully observed a senior resident perform a delicate procedure for hours. I was amazed by how stoic the mentoring surgeon was, and how closely he observed the resident.

---

[35] This includes patient care and not just isolating myself to study independently.

The surgeon demonstrated restraint—allowing the resident to do the procedure on his own and encouraging him along the way. The surgeon was tremendously patient; he had performed this surgical procedure thousands of times and surely would have been quicker than the resident if he performed it himself. But he knew he had to ensure that the next generation of surgeons were as good or better than his generation. It was his duty to teach, and he took it very seriously. Once the surgery was over, the attending surgeon sat with the resident and discussed his performance. He gave specific feedback on technical areas he needed to work on and complimented the resident's skills. I was impressed by this professional dynamic. It reminded me of Yoda training a jedi, the mentoring relationship was enviable. It was obvious that the mentoring surgeon had developed the trust of the resident, the resident was comfortable discussing his weaknesses with him.

Despite this experience, I soon realized I was not crazy about the operating room, even in the best environments. I was more energized and inspired by direct patient interaction rather than what I saw as the more *task*-based day-to-day of a surgeon.

I have great respect for the field of surgery, and I am grateful for their meaningful work. Most surgeons I met were kind, articulate, and encouraging. Sometimes, however, I was baffled by the behavior of some of the surgeons who I had envisioned as calm, cool, and assertive. For the most part they behaved like normal people. They wore their emotions on their sleeves. I often saw two versions of the same person—the one who stood in front of the patient and explained the surgery, and the one who hovered over the operating table and openly expressed emotions like frustration, rigidity, and cockiness. They were respectful speaking with the patient before the surgery and comforted patients and their families. But there was an air of paternalism and power the surgeons held over the surgical residents behind closed doors. It was not consistent with the vision I had of collaboration and virtue. Quickly my perceived magic of the OR faded and revealed a less idealistic reality: a cold, well-lit room where residents tried to perform a procedure while we all watched, the surgeon shouting commands throughout and ultimately taking over for the resident when it became clear it was not going to be done correctly or quickly enough. And then everyone moved on. Like a team of mechanics. And the culture among the residents and the attending surgeons was tense. It was a difficult environment for medical students to be in at times, since it felt like we had to agree with the surgeons and with the residents even when they oftentimes were at odds. We also had to always stay on our toes because during a surgery at any point the surgeon or a resident could drill you with questions about the procedure.[36] The questions could be technical, like "what is this layer of fascia called" or "why are we doing this procedure" or the questions could me more general like "what are the reasons for removing a gallbladder?"

One of the residents on this rotation took me under her wing. She always pulled me aside to teach me about the surgery and quizzed me on anatomical landmarks and pathophysiology to prepare me for the case. She regularly commented on how impressed she was with my knowledge and ability to explain my medical analysis. This was very encouraging to me. It made me feel good to think that I was performing well. She told me I had great unteachable manual skills and was

------

[36] This is called "pimping" in the medical world. Simply put, it is when a more senior medical professional asks a trainee questions relevant to the medical case.

impressed by my ability to suture and dress wounds. She said I had an "intuitive spatial awareness" that would serve me well in any specialty. She texted me encouraging messages after a 14-hour shift. She vented to me about how challenging the culture of surgery can be for her, and how she wished to return to her home state across the country. And I tried to offer her support, I expressed empathy and genuinely felt badly that a good person with great intentions was going through such a tough time on her path to be a surgeon.

When I received my evaluation, I discovered that this resident, someone who I considered a new friend, and had nominated for a resident teaching award, had given me by far the most brutal evaluation of my life.

Many of the things were outright false. She said I was underprepared, aloof, uninterested. That I was not helpful, and clearly did not care about surgery. She said I was impossible to teach because of this. At first, I thought it was a mistake, she had meant to evaluate someone else. But I learned this was not the case. I started to doubt myself—I wondered if I was not appropriately expressing myself to others I worked with. I wondered how I could better show my engagement in the OR, and how I could more effectively communicate my eagerness to learn. I wondered if my nervousness was interpreted as aloofness. I doubted some of the traits I am most proud of—that I always brought a positive attitude to the teams I worked with. I was confused and wanted to confront her, but never did. I figured no good could come of it, and I was so rattled I did not want to even harp on it any longer. I wanted to put the rotation behind me and focus on the next one. I regret not reaching out to her about it. I wish I could have gotten an explanation and some closure. But I felt powerless, and I doubted my own sanity—I wondered, did I read this entire relationship wrong?

Over time I have come to realize this resident likely put me down to make herself feel better. Perhaps she felt she was "paying it forward" because this was the harsh way she was evaluated when she was a medical student. Perhaps it makes her feel good to make it tough for others to achieve success. Maybe she knew I wouldn't be applying into surgery, so my evaluation didn't matter. It's also possible she truly believed the evaluation was accurate—that we had a miscommunication. I only wish this had been discussed in our feedback sessions prior to the evaluation. The psychology behind it is tough to parse out, but the power that evaluators have; the ability to control your future with a one-sided evaluation, is unfair. Unfortunately, these stories are not uncommon among my peers.

This experience gave me profound insight into how medical training can perpetuate a vicious system of belittling and offloading trauma onto the next generation.

The truth is that residents across all specialties work insane hours and are paid very little. Residents, who are full medical doctors and do most of the work at academic hospitals, are grossly underpaid and have little control or autonomy. For example, when medical students enroll in the residency match process, we must sign a document that relinquishes any possibility of negotiating our salaries. Surgical residents often work over 100 hours a week, and salaries typically are in the range of $60,000-$80,000 a year. It makes sense that some residents might feel dissatisfied and underappreciated in their job. I can understand that when someone feels a loss of control in their lives, they might seek it in other ways—by demanding medical students arrive at the hospital at impossibly early times for instance, or by evaluating them poorly.

Chapter VIII: Lessons from My First Patients

Juan

One late Friday afternoon on my general surgery rotation, the surgical case that I was assisting with was wrapping up. I glanced at the clock, and it was 5:15 pm, and so I wondered if this might be the last case of the day. A few minutes later, one of the residents entered the OR and asked me if I wanted to scrub in for the next case in the adjacent room. Thoughts of coming home before dinner to enjoy a quiet restful night with my wife evaporated, I agreed to join for the next surgery, expressing eagerness and appreciation for the opportunity.

It was a patient with a perirectal abscess that needed draining. The patient was a 33-year-old male, and I helped him onto the operating table and the anesthesiologist started working to put him under. I helped strap him safely to the operating table, which had become a skill I had learned quickly which helped me feel useful in the OR.

The resident and I propped his legs up in stirrups and cleaned the surgical area. There was a tennis ball sized firm red mass adjacent to the anus. The patient had the abscess for a couple of weeks. Understandably, despite the pain, the patient delayed seeking treatment in the hope that it would resolve on its own. Anal abscesses are not uncommon. The glands that are around the anus can become infected, and an abscess can form. Since an abscess is a walled-off infection, it's tough for oral antibiotics to penetrate the infection site. So, the treatment for abscesses, wherever they are on the body, is generally to do an incision and drainage. Usually, this can be done in the emergency room under local anesthetic. This case was a large abscess that seemed to be growing in a way that was obstructing the rectum, so within the OR, under general anesthesia, was the safest option for this case.

I really felt for the patient. He was only a few years older than me. Once it was time for the procedure, I stood beside the resident as she made an incision over the red bulge that abutted the patient's rectum. The next thing I knew a jet of thick white pus ejected through the air and onto the linoleum tile floor. It flowed freely and forcefully out of the incision for what seemed like a full 5 seconds. My gloves began to fill with cold sweat, and I suddenly felt a shiver. I looked around; I saw black spots. I was scrubbed in, fully gowned up in surgical gloves, gown, and cap. I took a wobbly step backwards. The attending glanced in my direction, "don't fall onto the surgical site" he stated firmly. Beneath me I felt a nurse placing a stool and pushing me down onto it from the shoulders. She pulled me away from the operating field and began ripping off my gown and fanning me with paper.

I was so grateful for her kindness and support. She anticipated what was happening and acted. She made me feel better. She told me that it was normal to feel lightheaded sometimes in the OR, and that I should get something to eat and drink. She told me that she used to feel the same way when she started. She told me not to let it influence my decision to become a surgeon if that is what I wanted. This small act of kindness was so meaningful for me on that day, and I won't ever forget what it felt like to be cared for in that way when I was in such a vulnerable position. I truly aspire to offer that same support to the future students who are on my team. I eventually made it home that night to enjoy a relaxing pasta dinner with my wife. But any sort of cream-sauce was off the menu.

Gerald

Patients who I met on the psychiatric inpatient ward
were endlessly fascinating to speak with. So many of
them have tremendous courage. Many patients with
schizophrenia, for example, oftentimes confront fear on
a regular basis during psychotic episodes. They have no
choice in the matter, and still they persevere.[37]

One of the patients who I spoke with had come to the
hospital because he was experiencing suicidal thoughts.
He was at home alone and was overcome with
depression and found himself contemplating a plan to
kill himself, so he chose to come to the emergency
psychiatric ward. The patient was in his mid-sixties and
had become accustomed to suicidal thoughts
throughout his life. He knew how to deal with the
situation, and he made the right choice to come to the
hospital.

Once he was seen in the emergency department, the
decision was made to admit the patient to the inpatient
psychiatric unit. Obviously, this is very disruptive to
the lives of patients. They don't know how long they
will be in the hospital and so must disconnect from
obligations for an unknown period. This includes
missing work without warning or may disrupt a

---

[37] Imagine how stressful the COVID-19 pandemic has
been for patients who are paranoid or schizophrenic.
Everyone is wearing masks, and they are being told that
a deadly disease can be spread rapidly that cannot be
seen by the naked eye. This 'invisible' disease requires
isolation to curb its spread. This combination of factors
can cause significant distress within this community of
patients, and it's important to consider when caring for
them.

patient's ability to care for others they are normally responsible for—like an elderly parent or a child.

This patient, Gerald, was upset that he was going to be admitted. He wanted to go home. He was worried that his boyfriend would be upset with him. He was concerned he was burdening others in his life to pick up his responsibilities.

I was explaining the clinical plan to the patient once we were on the wards. He sat across from me in a hospital gown. He asked me how long he would be in the hospital. I responded that the team and I think having him here for a few days, to assess how he is feeling on a new medication, would be appropriate.

The patient then grew irate—he wanted to leave immediately. He felt that he was being kept at the hospital against his will. He blamed me and shouted that I was being dishonest with him in the emergency department when I had not told him he would have to stay as an inpatient for so long. He wanted me to get the documents so that he could leave AMA (against medical advice). He shouted at me that I had tricked him.

I felt sad for Gerald that he was so agitated. I understood where he was coming from. He felt like he had no control of his life, and that can be a very scary situation to be in. I told Gerald that he could absolutely leave whenever he likes, and I would fill out the documents if that is what he wants. This put Gerald at ease a bit. The last thing I wanted for him was to feel trapped. I didn't want him to hesitate if he needed to come to the hospital again. I then asked him what I could do to put his mind at ease a bit about the responsibilities he has to take care of at home over the next few days. He mentioned that he wanted to get on the "right medications" so that he did not have to come back into the hospital anytime soon. I told him that was our goal too.

He mentioned to me that he has a dog at home, and he wants to call his neighbor to ask him to feed the dog and walk her while he's in the hospital. I said that I would be happy to retrieve his phone (which was confiscated when he was admitted to the inpatient psychiatric floor) and help him reach out to the neighbor. The patient stared silently—he seemed to be wondering if he should stay at the hospital or continue to request leaving AMA.

I asked him, what type of dog do you have? He mentioned that he had a Pitbull terrier, and that she was the sweetest dog in the world. His expression softened a bit. I asked if I could see a picture of his dog on his phone—once I grab it for him to reach out to the neighbor. I told him that my wife and I had just adopted a Pitbull mix. He asked to see a picture and I pulled up several on my phone to show him. His manner completely changed. It no longer felt like a student doctor and a patient speaking on an inpatient psychiatric ward. It felt like two people discussing their dogs at a coffee shop. The patient was so lovely to speak with. Once I gave him his phone and he was able to contact the neighbor and ensure that his dog would be taken care of, he was visibly relieved. He thanked me profusely and agreed to stay at the hospital until his medications were adjusted appropriately. He and I continued to have a friendly relationship the rest of the time he was in the hospital. He even requested to speak to *only* me as his doctor, and when I was out over the weekend, he asked when I would be back. Going from screaming in my face, calling me a liar, and requesting to be discharged only a few days prior to developing this trusted patient-doctor relationship with the patient was deeply gratifying.

From this experience I learned that showing your own personality and connecting with patients in a real human-to-human way, rather than a strict paternalistic relationship, can go a long way in putting a patient at ease and ultimately leads to better patient care and outcomes. After caring for the patient for a few days and he was discharged, he left me a letter thanking me for my kindness and wishing me well. This experience also reminded me that when patients come to the hospital, it is not a good day for them to say the least. They are stressed out and their daily routine is disrupted. It is important to remember that, to cut them slack and allow for emotional reactions. It is important to not take things personally in the hospital, and that making patients feel comfortable and heard is incredibly important.

<u>Samantha</u>

Throughout 3rd year, medical students are often faced with unique and complex ethical decisions for the first time. During my neurology rotation I was on an evening shift with the team that takes care of stroke patients. We were paged to the emergency department to see a 25-year-old female who presented with complaints of numbness in her left leg. She was a nurse within the hospital system. When we saw the patient, she was in no pain or distress that was apparent to me. But she did state that she suddenly lost feeling in her entire leg.

I performed a test of her sensation and the patient reported that she was unable to feel touch in any area of the right leg, but she reported no other sensory deficits throughout her body. She also reported that she could not move her left leg at all—a motor deficit in a specific region would raise suspicion for a stroke.

She told me that she is anemic and was getting a bone marrow biopsy in the hospital when this happened. I was worried for the patient. I thought maybe a nerve was damaged when the bone marrow biopsy was taken. Or I considered the possibility of a brain bleed that was unrelated to the procedure she got in the hospital. I also wondered why such a seemingly healthy young patient would need a bone marrow biopsy in the first place.

After seeing the patient, I reviewed her chart further. Apparently, she had a history of showing up to hospitals with bizarre complaints. On one occasion, the patient underwent a colonoscopy because of her low red blood cell counts. One potential reason for anemia might be bleeding from the GI tract, and so an endoscopy and colonoscopy is a reasonable test to assess for bleeding. GI bleeding must be ruled out early because it can be life-threatening. On colonoscopy, shards of glass were discovered in the colon. The patient had been consuming glass. On another occasion, there was a note in the patient's chart where the clinician had written about the possibility that the patient was drawing her own blood, which would cause her to become anemic on lab testing. This condition of inflicting medical harm on oneself is known as factitious disorder or Munchausen's syndrome.

I had read about this condition in medical textbooks. Many people have heard of this disorder because it has been prominently featured on various medical tv series. I recalled a specific episode of a show that I had watched where the character in the story was inflicting medical harm on her daughter—which is known as factitious disorder imposed on another or—Munchausen by proxy. When asked to identify patients on written board exams who might have factitious disorder; the stereotypical patient in the question stem was a young female patient who worked in the health care field and who might have access to medications or medical devices like phlebotomy needles. This was, as they say in the hospital, a textbook case of factitious disorder. My evening shift was ending, so I presented the case to the neurology resident who was taking over for the rest of the night. This happened to be my last shift of the rotation, so I would not follow the patient anymore and I shifted focus to my next rotation the next day. But the case was memorable to me. I had a visceral reaction to picturing the patient swallowing glass. I hoped she got the psychiatric care she needed to deal with these impulses. My note in her chart outlined this entire picture for the next doctor, and I articulated my concern to my attending.

Several months later, I was on a night rotation in the pediatric emergency department at a different hospital. I saw the woman who was my former patient working on the floors. She was the nurse for my pediatric patient who came in with an upper respiratory virus called Croup. It was a strange feeling to see my former patient working in the medical setting, taking care of children. I wondered if she recognized me. Admittedly, I also wondered if she should be caring for such vulnerable and delicate patients. I wondered if I would want my child's nurse to be actively struggling with such severe mental health issues. I wondered if the hospital staff even knew that the young pediatric nurse often drained her own blood with hospital supplies and admitted herself to different hospitals throughout the city. I wondered if she did this during her shifts. I didn't know what to do. I wondered if I should have followed up with the patient even after the rotation had ended. I wondered if I was even allowed to do this as a student doctor. What constitutes a HIPPA[38] violation in this circumstance?

---

[38] Health Insurance Portability and Accountability Act of 1996—stipulates that any personally identifiable information that is attained in healthcare setting is

Ultimately, I assured myself that the nurses are closely monitored by the rest of the team. And hoped she sought mental health care since I saw her in the emergency department as a patient. I wondered what my role was in this ethical quandary. Was I ethically required to work with a different nurse and see a new patient? Should I have checked her medical records to see if she sought the psychiatric care she needed? These questions still linger on my mind today. My decision was based on my sense that we are not cops and caring for a patient in the hospital once does not grant a student doctor the right (or even ability) to determine their professional life.

Rudy

On my family medicine rotation, I enjoyed being able to have longer appointments with patients in the outpatient clinic. My rotation occurred early on in my third year and so seeing patients on my own was relatively new to me, but I was eager to speak to patients in person—even if it required wearing a mask and face shield.

One patient was a middle-aged man who was a Taxi driver in Manhattan. He originally was from Nigeria and had been living in New York City for 15 years. Before seeing the patient, the attending physician told me that the patient can be difficult about agreeing to make lifestyle changes to keep his blood sugar under control.

---

protected. It's a federal law that created national standards to protect sensitive patient information from being disclosed without the patient's consent or knowledge.

Despite the warning from the physician, I really enjoyed speaking with the affable man who entered the exam room. He was charming and wanted to get to know me on a personal level. With the benefit of a short patient-list that day, I was able to fully engage with him and discuss his upbringing and family he has nearby and family back in Nigeria. We discussed his favorite football teams. This relationship-forming part of the visit was fun for me, it is one of the most important reasons I wanted to become a doctor in the first place and contributed to my decision to pursue a residency in internal medicine. I enjoy the personal interaction that medical care allows for, and I believe that forming a relationship with patients allows for mutual trust and ultimately allows for more effective patient care.

Eventually, I steered the conversation to discuss his health. He gained some weight over the pandemic, and his hemoglobin A1C[39] levels were elevated from his last visit. We discussed ways in which he can improve his lifestyle and eating habits to reach attainable goals for his weight and blood-sugar. He seemed eager and motivated to make changes in his diet and with exercise.

---

[39] Measuring the hemoglobin A1C level is a test that tells you a patient's average level of blood sugar over a three-month period. Hemoglobin is the iron-containing oxygen transport protein in red blood cells. *Glycated* hemoglobin is a form of hemoglobin that is chemically linked to sugar. Hemoglobin is a sticky molecule— most sugars including glucose and fructose bind with hemoglobin when present in the bloodstream. A normal A1C level is below 5.7%, a level of 5.7%-6.4% indicates prediabetes, and a level of 6.5% or more indicates diabetes.

One of the most touching moments I experienced in medical school occurred at the end of the patient interaction, when the patient asked me if I could be his primary doctor moving forward. He wanted to see me in the clinic for his next appointment.

This question was so validating to me. In just one meeting the patient felt he could trust me. He wanted to work with me to improve his health, and that was incredibly moving. I am grateful for this patient experience because it made me feel like my instincts as a future doctor were effective. I learned from this interaction how powerful it can be to take your time with patients and get to know them on a personal level before delving into health recommendations and plans for improvement.

Chapter IX: 4th year

Once clerkships are completed, medical students typically have decided what specialty they wish to pursue. During this time, it is important for students to do formal rotations in the specialty of their choosing. This roughly entails a month working on the same team in the hospital, taking on the role of a first-year resident (aka intern).[40] Most students are looking for letters of recommendation from attendings on these rotations. In some smaller sub-specialties, building connections is important and if students develop a relationship with an attending it can go a long way. There is some variability as to how 4th year is structured based on the specialty; for some residency programs it is common that students do what is called an "away rotation."[41]

The sub-internships are the first-time medical students are meant to take full ownership over their patients. That includes placing orders for medications in the electronic medical record (EMR) (that must be approved by the resident before going through to the pharmacy), speaking with patients and their families, and responding to their pager about any urgent issues regarding their patients. It is an exciting time. It is the first time we are seeing firsthand what it will be like to be a resident, and the rest of the team expects the sub-intern to be working at the resident level.

---

[40] It was shocking to me to learn that after years of training and finally obtaining an MD, the first year as a doctor you are an 'intern.' One of many ways medical training effectively keeps your ego in check! And as a 4th-year on rotations you hold the glamorous title of "*sub*-intern" abbreviated "Sub-I."

[41] This is common in emergency medicine, general surgery, and surgical subspecialties like otorhinolaryngology (ENT), orthopedics, or plastic surgery.

During my first sub-internship in internal medicine, I was struck by the importance of team culture. The inpatient medicine teams are comprised of an attending, a junior resident or senior resident, two first-year residents, and the sub-intern (me).[42] The teams typically changed every two weeks, so over the course of my four weeks on the rotation I was a part of three different teams. I joined the first team in their second week on the service. The senior resident set the tone of the group—she assumed the leadership role on the team. On my first morning I introduced myself to the group. The resident paused rounds to ask me several introductory questions in front of the group. She asked me where I am from, what specialty I am applying into for residency, and she explained what some of the expectations are for a sub-intern. She encouraged me that everyone on the team will be available for my questions and that they all want to help me along the way. She said that if I am ever uncomfortable or doing tasks that I feel I should not be doing to let her know directly. She said I should only be focusing on my patients, that I am not there to do menial tasks (aka 'scut work'). The rest of the team nodded approvingly throughout this quick orientation. It made me feel included and important to the group.

This culture of inclusion resulted in more educational rounds; everyone was speaking on rounds—asking questions during patient presentations. It was clear everyone was paying close attention to each patient presentation. Throughout the day each person checked in on each other's patients and was eager to help. When

---

[42] Residents are often distinguished by their year of training "post-graduation" from medical school. So, an intern is a "PGY1." For internal medicine residency, which is three years in duration, a junior resident is referred to as a PGY2, and a senior resident is a PGY3.

there were disagreements about treatment plans, the attending physician did not defiantly declare her plan as the only option. It did not feel like a hierarchy, everyone felt like colleagues. There was mutual respect, and this made me eager to come into the hospital each day.

My next team could not have been more different. On the first day, my new group rounded in a small conference room. Without introductions we dove right in, presenting the patients on the list from top to bottom. Each patient presentation was a one-on-one conversation between the attending and the resident who was covering the patient. A short time into rounds one of the interns typed on his laptop as we all sat around the conference table listening to another resident present a patient. Without warning, the attending shot a disapproving look at the intern, and she exclaimed, "don't write your notes during rounds." The intern closed his laptop quietly as we moved on to the next patient.

When it was my turn to present, I was very nervous. I did not want to miss a key detail in my presentation, I worried about talking too much, giving too much background that the attending did not want. The attending had cut-off the previous presentations early on, instead bombarding the resident with questions about lab results. If they didn't know one off the top of their head, she would shake her head disapprovingly.

I started presenting, "This patient is a 49-year-old Female with…" The attending cut me off. The intern had opened his laptop again and started typing. She turned to him and said, "what are you typing?" The intern said, "Oh I'm not writing notes. I'm looking something up." The attending turned to me to continue and so I began to speak again. Immediately I was cut off by the attending. She turned back to the intern, "what are you looking up?" The intern fumbled through an answer and appeared to be frantic on the laptop. The attending turned her head to see what was on his laptop. She said, "I told you not to write notes during rounds." We sat in silence for a moment as the attending sat seething in her seat. She turned to me, forced a smile to mask her anger, and nodded indicating I should continue my presentation.

This was not the team environment that was conducive to asking questions, being vulnerable, and learning. It felt like torture getting through rounds every day. The attending spoke the most in the group by far. This culture permeated throughout the group. The residents seemed to work in parallel, not often communicating. There were mistakes—medications were ordered late; labs were not drawn appropriately. It was miserable to work in that type of environment. My days went by slowly and I even began to doubt my chosen specialty.

Leaders in a group determine the culture of the team. It is important to build safety for the team members, to design a culture of belonging. Effective communication relies on cooperation and mutual respect. In medicine which has a deep-seated culture of hierarchy, it is especially important for leaders to aggressively combat an egocentric group dynamic.

4th year is also a time when students participate in elective rotations. One of my first elective rotations was on the medical oncology consult service. Whenever the primary team taking care of a patient wants to get the opinion of an oncologist, they would page us to see the patient. This includes patients who come into the emergency department with 'non-specific' symptoms like unintentional weight loss, fever, sweatiness, cough, or fatigue. These symptoms, coupled with imaging or lab tests consistent with possible cancer would warrant a call to the oncology consult service. Another example might be a patient with a known history of cancer who is in the hospital for another reason, like pneumonia, and the primary team wants to know what medications to pause or avoid due to the history of cancer.

One patient we were called to see deeply affected me. Mrs. R, a 39-year-old female with late-stage gastric cancer, had spent the last month in a different hospital and was eventually told that there was nothing more that could be done for her—they wanted to send her home to die. The patient and her husband were not satisfied with this, so they asked to be transferred to our hospital. When I saw this patient, she was shockingly young. I couldn't believe she was only 10 years older than me. Typically, the patients I would see on this service were in their 60s, 70s, or 80s—cancer is more common in these age demographics as it typically occurs because of decades of cell turn-over.[43] This young woman was in visible pain. She was groaning and clutching her belly. She couldn't move much, and she spoke to me in a low whisper.

When we got to talking, she told me about her three daughters—her youngest was 18 months old and Mrs. R wanted to make it to see her second birthday. It was

---

[43] Cells in your body are constantly replicating and re-generating. Your skin cells, for example, regenerate approximately every four weeks. After decades of what we call "cell turnover" there can be replication mistakes that occur on the molecular level that can cause problems. These problems can be a result of cellular damage, like from carcinogens in cigarette smoke or from UV radiation from years of getting too much unprotected sun exposure. There are certain proteins that act as *safety* breaks for cellular replication, but they can faulter and stop effectively doing their job—this might result in an over-proliferation of cell growth resulting in cancer.

heartbreaking to hear about Mrs. R's life. She had such young kids, and I could not imagine the emotional pain Mrs. R felt realizing she would not be around to see them grow up. She repeated the phrase to me, "I know I'm going to die, and dying hurts and that's okay." I kept responding that she shouldn't be in this much pain and that my team would adjust her pain medication to make her more comfortable. She simply nodded in response. Later, only after leaving her room, did I realize that while she was in physical pain from the cancer and the surgeries, the pain she was describing to me was not one that could be treated with pain medicine. It was the slow realization and understanding of what she was leaving behind.

Mrs. R had multiple surgeries for her stomach tumors, which had metastasized throughout her intestines and abdominal cavity—she had multiple tubes in her stomach that were draining abscesses that had developed because of the surgeries. She also had an open surgical wound that spanned roughly 8 inches in the midline of her abdomen. This wound had opened ripping through her stitches, and a surgical bag was placed over it to prevent infection and foreign material from entering her abdomen. The patient asked me if I could close the wound. I told her I would speak with the surgical team about doing that.

I felt angry on behalf of my patient. Why was she left in this state for so long? Why didn't the surgical team close this wound in her belly? If I had a wound like that, I would feel unsafe and scared. I would not feel myself; I would feel un-whole. The surgery team said that they couldn't close the wound because it might risk infection, and that because of her decreased ability to form scar tissue due to the chemotherapy and cancer, the sutured wound would not heal. Essentially the general oncology surgeons were telling me that there was nothing that they planned to do for the patient. She just needed pain medication and to be released home. I remember feeling my skin turn hot, like when you're a passenger in a car and someone just slammed on the breaks to avoid a crash. I then felt nauseous. I realized I would have to relay this information to my patient.

I have often felt dissatisfied with how doctors deal with end-of-life care. When your mind is fully aware of imminent death, what tools do we provide to help patients grapple with this scary and profoundly sad time? This aspect of caring for people seems like a crucial component to treating the 'whole patient,' as we were all taught in medical school. This experience further solidified my decision to care for terminally ill patients. I hope to be an Oncologist that deals with end-of-life care with the same sensitivity and attention called upon when delivering bad news about a new diagnosis, or when outlining a complex treatment plan with the patient and their family. It is an essential part of our job as doctors and should be embraced as an opportunity to help patients live their last days in the way *they* want.

Chapter X: What to do when faced with challenges?

When you start medical school, you give up a lot of control of your life. You sacrifice your time and money and forego other opportunities that would allow you to live a more 'normal' life.

Although I lived in Manhattan during medical school, which is where most of my friends also lived, I had to pass up most parties. I had to say no to bachelor parties and weeknight social gatherings. I had to show up late to engagement parties in my scrubs and I had to leave early from family weekend vacations. This can be frustrating, and it's important to have tools in place to cope.

Build in time for yourself each day
My biology professor in college is a very charismatic and wise man who is a clear and creative thinker. Once when I visited during his office hours, he could tell I was stressed with finals approaching. Instead of offering generic advice he told me: appreciate living your life in chaotic bursts of energy. He said that one thing he liked about being a student was that you would study hard for weeks leading up to an exam, then there was immediate relief, and you could relax. Your job as a student is simple, to ride the intensity upswings of focus and intense learning and studying, but it is also your job to ride the trough on the activity curve. Simply exist as an enthusiastic passenger on this ride and do not fight it. Life will be a lot more enjoyable if you can achieve this Zen way of thinking.

Don't take yourself too seriously
During my third-year obstetrics and gynecology clerkship I was fortunate to be paired with my friend Archie. On our first day of the rotation, we met one of

our residents named Sydney. We introduced ourselves and her first question was: can I use one of your otoscopes to see my patient? Archie and I laughed. We thought she was joking. When Sydney stood silently staring at us, we realized she was serious.

At this point I worried I was making a poor first impression and I wondered if Sydney thought we were ill-prepared for the clerkship. I wondered if she would evaluate me and write that I did not bring the proper instruments to the wards. I wondered if other students always carried otoscopes around.

An otoscope is a very specific instrument used to examine ear canals. They are the instruments that hang on the walls of most medical exam rooms, the ones that are capped with the plastic cone before a doctor looks in your ear. I had never seen any medical student carrying around an otoscope. Owning one seemed absurd to me. On top of that, we were on our obstetrics and gynecology rotation, which to my knowledge did not really have much to do with the ear canals. Archie and I looked at each other and responded that we did not have an otoscope on us. She was visibly disappointed and informed us that she had carried one as a medical student and we should do the same.

Every interaction with residents and attendings seems to carry a lot of weight on rotations. I couldn't help but think, "this person will be grading us, how can I recover from this?" But I also wondered if it would be wasted energy to bend over backwards trying to satisfy Sydney's every wish. My experiences told me that some residents were never satisfied, no matter how hard you worked or how much time you spent at the hospital, you would never get their approval. I realized that relying on external factors for *my* self-worth was a dangerous precedent to set for myself. Archie and I were on the same page. We knew we might not be getting the best evaluation from her at this point, and probably did not have much of a shot at a glowing review no matter what we did.

Neither of us ended up purchasing an otoscope.

Later in the week, Archie and I were scheduled to deliver our individual presentations to the rest of the clerks on the OB/GYN rotation and to the two clerkship site leaders. Archie was assigned to work with Sydney that day and spent the morning with her; but once a week we had scheduled lunch presentations with our site leaders. As we are sitting in the conference room, Archie began his presentation, going over a case from earlier in the week and teaching surgical concepts based on the case. No more than two minutes into his presentation, Sydney walked by the room where he was presenting and interrupted, saying directly to Archie in front of the entire group "why aren't you in the OR?" He responded, "Oh, I'm sorry, I thought the next case did not start for another hour or so and today is my presentation which I'm giving right now."

Sydney responded that he should be in the OR right now prepping the room.[44] Archie apologized to the group, changed into scrubs, and went up to the OR.

---

[44] The job of a 3rd year medical student is always very ambiguous. Each resident and attending has different expectations. Keep in mind, as a 3rd year medical student we are paying full tuition (over $30,000 a semester at my school). Our daily job is our education. Some residents and attendings take advantage of our being there and ask us to do menial tasks. For example, I spent an hour moving chairs during my OB/GYN rotation. When someone who is grading you asks you to do something, you drop what you are doing and do it. Even if you may be in the middle of a presentation.

When he got there Sydney asked him if he had introduced himself to the patient yet.

Archie responded, "No I didn't have a chance since I thought the next surgery was scheduled for an hour from now and I was delivering my presentation today."

Sydney responded that this was unacceptable, and that if Archie wanted to be in the OR he had to introduce himself to the patient first. So, Archie rushed to the perioperative area where he could find the patient to introduce himself. The patient had a mask on and was being anesthetized when he entered her room.

"Hi I'm Archie, a 3rd year medical student who is part of the surgical team. I'll be in the OR during your surgery. We'll take good care of you today."

This patient obviously couldn't respond. She was going under, actively getting anesthetized for the surgery. She could not even speak with the mask on that was delivering a sedative. The anesthesiologist simply looked at Archie with befuddlement.

I felt badly for Archie. One might wonder why he didn't stick up for himself when he was interrupted during his presentation.

Why not respond to Sydney, "I'm actually supposed to deliver this presentation right now, I'm sorry for the misunderstanding and appreciate you allowing me to scrub in but will have to catch the next surgery."

But he did not speak up and neither did any of the other medical students in the room including myself. I couldn't believe how rude Sydney was, how she must have viewed us as subordinates who would never complain or disobey her orders. I even wondered if she was abused in the same way when she was a medical student and did not know how else to work with students.

Later, when Archie explained to me what happened with the patient, we laughed at the ridiculous situation. Archie, a personable and highly sensitive person with a great bedside manner, was put in an impossible situation—one in which he felt the only way out was to carry out absurd orders. Despite our laughs, I am sure being forced to behave in a nonsensical way worried that he was making the patient uncomfortable made Archie feel awful. The experience of powerlessness and humiliation inflicts deep wounds.

The next day Archie and I arrived at the hospital at 6:20 am. We both discussed getting to the hospital early, we wanted to give our biggest effort so that even if our resident did not appreciate us, we still would know we did the right thing and did not give up. The residents typically arrived at 7:00 and began rounding on patients at 7:15.

Archie and I got there early to review the surgeries that would be occurring that day so that we could be prepared for the flurry of questions that would be floated our way in the operating room like: "why are we doing this operation?" or "what is the most common complication of the operation we are doing today?" We worked in the medical student lounge, which was in the basement of the hospital, down the hall from the resident lounge. There was a computer in our lounge, and we looked up the patients and quizzed each other on the cases to prepare for the long morning ahead.

We kept poking our heads out of the medical student lounge to see when the residents would arrive so we could join them. Typically, the intern texted us when they were about to head upstairs for rounds. At 7:00 on the dot we walked over to the resident lounge since we did not want to take the chance of missing them, but it was locked, and the lights were off. At 7:01 am (I know this because my texts were time-stamped) I texted Sydney asking if they were around. She responded, "we're rounding." Archie and I sprinted up to the 7th floor where gynecology rounds occurred. We walked into the patient room where they were rounding at 7:04 a bit out of breath, sweating, but in good spirits. I wanted to slip into the room quietly without distracting the patient and planned on apologizing to the residents for being late after leaving the patient's room. I knew it would not be best to try to explain that we were here early preparing for the days' surgeries.

The patient happened to be a woman who we both spent time with the previous day. As we entered the room, she excitedly acknowledged us "Oh yay! My guys are here this morning. I was hoping you would be here today; I need your good energy the day of my surgery." Sydney was in the middle of a physical examination, and I knew this would not bode well for us. The patient carried on "these guys are great, right?" speaking to Sydney and the other two residents in the room. I knew that we were in trouble, this reaction probably was the last thing that Sydney wanted to be a part of. I tried to alleviate the tenseness in the room, "oh stop it, you're the one who is great! It's always such a pleasure to see you," I responded so that Sydney didn't have to. Archie picked up what I was putting down and added "Now Mrs. Sutherland, are there any questions Adam or I can answer for you this morning?" I could tell Sydney was even more irritated than usual, I'd like to think she was checking Mrs. Sutherland's reflexes at this point and smashed the reflex hammer a bit too hard out of anger, grinding her teeth to the gums.

"No, no, I have the utmost trust in you two young fellas. What promising future doctors you both are. I'm so glad you're here."

We exited the room. Sydney pulled us aside, far from any patient room. This would be the first and only time I was yelled at by a resident throughout medical school. Ultimately, I remember feeling badly for Sydney—it seemed so easy to tap into her inner rage. She was seething. I was worried the nurses walking in and out of patient rooms around us were staring. I could feel my face getting warm with embarrassment.

"You two cannot be late again! How could you get to the hospital so late?[45] You should never come into a room when important information is being gathered from the patient. For the duration of the rotation, you are expected to pre-round on every single patient on the operating list before the residents.[46] You did that for your medicine rotation, you did that for your surgery rotation, there is no reason why you shouldn't do that for OB/GYN."[47] This last sentence was very telling me. It was obvious that Sydney had a chip on her shoulder

---

[45] As I mentioned previously, we arrived at the hospital 40 minutes before Sydney and the team of daytime residents.

[46] This was never the expectation for the rotation, and on the first day with a new team I always asked what the expectations were for 3rd year medical students. Again, to be clear, this is the first time I was hearing this.

[47] Neither of us pre-rounded before the residents on any rotation. This would mean waking the patients up from 5:30-6:00 before the residents woke them up from 7:15-9:00 to perform the same exact physical exam and ask for any overnight events. It's redundancy for punishments sake and ultimately the patient suffers from having further disruptions to their sleep for no benefit. Also, Archie had an overly eager co-3rd year medical student pre-round on patients once on a previous rotation and was yelled at for doing so.

and clearly thought: "Why wouldn't you treat this rotation like the other 'important ones'?" Sydney was interpreting our lateness as disrespectful to the rotation, to the specialty, and to her personally.

The false stereotype regarding gynecologists that I had heard numerous times on my general surgery rotation is that they are 'not real surgeons.' This perspective is rooted in sexism no doubt and is completely unfair. I once scrubbed into a urology surgery and the urologist disparaged urogynecologists[48] regularly saying, 'it's not a real specialty.' Medicine folks criticize OB/GYN doctors for consulting them for any medical issue, in their view even the most minor questions. The field of medicine is focused on prestige and appeal and insecurity can be a very powerful driver of behavior and self-worth. These were the thoughts going through my mind as Sydney admonished Archie and me.

I tell the story of Sydney because a different medical student in a different environment could have reacted in a much more detrimental way to this abuse. I did not internalize this unfounded criticism. Because I had Archie with me, and because I knew that this was more about Sydney than it was either of us, I was able to brush it off. This is something all medical students should learn early, and I am grateful I did. The more you rely on external affirmation for self-worth in

---

[48] Urology is a surgical subspecialty; trainees enter urology residency straight after medical school and spend at least 5 years in the operating room performing complex surgeries on the male and female urogenital system. Urogynecology is a subspecialty after OB/GYN residency that deals with the female urogenital system, typically dealing with conditions like stress incontinence—which might happen when physical movement or activity such as coughing puts pressure on the bladder, causing a leakage of urine.

medicine the more you are setting yourself up for
misery, and the more vulnerable you are to be abused
by the system. Medicine preys on the insecure and
eager-to-please. I kept reminding myself throughout the
tougher times in my rotations that: the patient should
always be the focus of my energy. It served as the
melodic mantra of my clinical years in medical school.

Practice Mindfulness Meditation

Two books greatly inform my practice of meditation
and mindfulness. "Mindfulness in Plain English," by
Henepola Gunaratana is an excellent introduction to
these concepts. "The Miracle of Mindfulness," by
Thich Nhat Hanh is also accessible, clear, and inspiring.

Mindfulness is the practice of being aware of your
feelings, emotions, or sensations. It is done by simply
observing them without judgement or interpretation. It
is a powerful way to focus on the present moment and
to live more fully. By practicing mindfulness, we can
live within the present moment. Our attention improves
and we become more focused. We listen more
effectively, and we enable ourselves to enjoy the beauty
of the now. With an increased attention and awareness,
we become more connected to those around us and
more generous and compassionate. We see daily
frustrations for what they are rather than building them
up, we note them and move on with our day. We aren't
shackled by our emotions. If we are irritated, we accept
that. If we are joyous, we accept that too.

There are many ways to practice being mindful.
Mindfulness meditation, setting aside time to simply sit
in a quiet space to meditate and observe emotions as
they flow through your mind, is one way to hone the
skill of mindfulness. Meditation is the process of
cultivating mindfulness, and once it is cultivated it must

be practiced throughout your normal daily routine. Practice mindfulness when doing a task like washing the dishes or making the bed. Practice mindfulness when listening to a patient, reviewing lab results on epic, or walking through the halls of the hospital. You can practice mindfulness by simply focusing on your breath. Mindfulness trains us to bring full awareness to whatever we are doing right now.

Without a mindfulness practice, from the moment many of us awake in the morning, our mind begins to think about what must get done that day. When we get to the hospital we listen to sign-out about our new patients, figuring out what we must do afterward before rounds begin later that morning. We might rush through our patient lists, checking on them, asking the questions we know our attendings might ask later instead of focusing on the patient with our own eyes and ears in that moment. We make calls to consult services to check on a patient. We may feel frustrated and angry if the consulting doctor resists. We finish our to-do list before the attending arrives for rounds and we feel relief. We take this time to scroll through our phones, thinking about our plans for our day off in 4 days—longing for that time to catch-up on sleep, see friends, and eat delicious food. In a sense, our minds and our days are not our own. We never actually live in the present moment. When practicing mindfulness in the hospital, we become more focused on patients, and more tuned in to what they are feeling and saying. We listen more closely, ask better questions, and because we are not focused on distractions—we have a stronger memory of our interactions with patients. We also are aware of any non-verbal communication that may be occurring. We create better connections with our colleagues.

Medical school applicants are not strangers to planning. We are constantly expected to look to the future. In College we fantasized about our medical school prospects. We rounded out our applications by participating in research, volunteer activities, attaining leadership roles, and extracurriculars. We studied to ensure that we performed well on standardized exams. We went to lectures to get good grades; we took courses to boost our GPA.

In medical school we go through our clinical rotations wondering, is this the right specialty for me? Would I be happy doing this as a career? Would I be a competitive applicant in this field? We scrutinize over details in residency programs, ranking from top to bottom our preferences. Would I want to live there for the next few years? How can I properly position myself for fellowships? Where would I get my morning coffee?

Being mindful can serve as the antidote for many of these harmful habits we have fallen into over the years. There is no better time than now to embark on your journey in mindfulness meditation. I am no expert on the ancient practice of meditation. From my readings and experience I structure my meditation sessions simply. Below I have outlined my sessions in eight steps. I hope it is helpful for some of you in starting your practice and eventually determining the structure that is best for you.

Step 1: Decide to sit for a specific, pre-determined amount of time. I sit for 30 minutes, but I started with 10 minutes.

Step 2: Find a quiet and comfortable place to sit. I like to sit cross-legged, but there are many different seated positions that people like to use. I like to sit in a position that makes me feel grounded and sturdy. I don't like to sit in a position that is too comfortable in case I am tempted to fall asleep. I bring a watch to place within eyesight because I don't want to use my phone, in case I get distracting messages or emails. I try to not be hyper-focused on the time and will not look at it until I think it has been close to 30 minutes since I began.

Step 3: Close your eyes and place your attention on your breath. Focus on the sensation of your breath, you can count your inhalations and exhalations up to ten, and then start over. You can inhale for four seconds, hold for four seconds, and release, counting for four seconds. This is called 'boxed' breathing. I like to inhale for a count of three, then exhale counting to eight. You can find many other breathing exercises or make up your own.

Step 4: Once I have paid attention to my breath, I then scan my body and notice any sensations. I might note stiffness in my back, or a hunger pang. I scan from my head to my toes and simply bring awareness to my body. I imagine I have a spotlight and use it to scan different areas of my body.

Step 5: I focus on my mind. I observe thoughts as they come and go. I note any emotions I am feeling that day. I picture myself sitting at a train station, observing trains as they whoosh by. I simply observe the thoughts come and go. If I become distracted, I bring my attention back to my breath, then back to my thoughts. It's important to try to *observe* your thoughts, rather than be *thinking* your thoughts. If you sense you're stuck in your thoughts, try to step back, and focus on your breath again. You don't want to be *on* the *traveling train*. Instead, try to stay on the *platform*, merely *aware* of the train coming and going.

Step 6: Once I am ready to move on, I gently remove myself from the train station in my mind and begin to think about things that I am grateful for. I list them in my mind. These things might seem silly and mundane like, I am thankful for my new shoes that give me stability and comfort throughout the day. Or I am thankful I was able to go for a run this morning. I also think of bigger things I am thankful for, like my wife and my family.

Step 7: I like to incorporate some visualization into my meditation practice. This can be something big that is coming up later in the week like, for example, a presentation. I like to visualize what it might feel like to stand up to deliver my presentation, I think about what people might get out of the presentation and I might consider what I want them to take away from it. The object of your visualization could also be something fun that is coming up like a vacation. Visualize what sensations you might feel when packing for your trip, and when landing at your destination. I try to stay away from fantasy visualizations, like accepting an award, because in most cases this can result in the ego running free.

Step 8: When it is time to end the meditation, I gently open my eyes and slowly and deliberately stretch out my legs and arms rising to a stand—ready to apply the mindfulness I have just cultivated throughout the rest of my day.

Afterward

Being mindful in the hospital helps me be a better doctor. Whether it's dealing with an irrational resident or grappling with the ethical challenges when seeing a new patient, ultimately, I remind myself of my mantra *'patient should be my focus.'* With the help of friends, I was able to take unfair criticism in stride and make funny and memorable experiences with them. In relation to Sydney, when we can view adversaries with empathy, we better understand their motivations and are slower to anger and frustration. When I was about to pass out in the OR, the nurse in the room viewed me with empathy and understanding. Instead of becoming annoyed or flustered—concerned I might delay the procedure or distract the surgeon—she showed me compassion, which deeply affected me in a positive way. When Gerald threw insults at me, instead of viewing him as an adversary or becoming offended, I was able to consider his struggles, and this enabled us to create a physician-patient bond moving forward built on the foundation of understanding and acceptance. These are the lessons that will stick with me from my first experiences in the hospital.

After I graduated from college, majoring in English literature, I started a program to take the science courses required to apply to medical school. I didn't come to the realization that I wanted to be a doctor until Senior year at WashU in St. Louis, and so after graduating, I started the formal pre-medical postbaccalaureate program at NYU. It's a 2-year program where students take General Chemistry, Biology, Biochemistry, Physics, Organic Chemistry, and the medical school entrance exam—the MCAT. I remember starting in Biology I the first semester—I hadn't taken any science courses since high school. We were thrown into the large undergraduate lecture at NYU, among hundreds of students who had just taken

AP biology months before. In those first months I was completely lost. I listened to recordings of the lecture on 0.5x speed and transcribed the lecture by hand to learn the material. I had to look up most of what I was writing down. It was an arduous process—a time filled with self-doubt.

Looking back on that time, now about to embark on my residency journey—feelings of self-doubt are not too foreign to me. I have felt alone at times throughout this process because it seemed like the students around me were *only* succeeding. But this is undoubtedly not the case. We all will face adversity at times, but we all will also succeed. It is okay to struggle, and it is okay to share it with your peers. Because often, they are dealing with similar feelings. And the best way to confront them is together, not in isolation.

About the Author:

Adam Ephraim graduated from Washington University in St. Louis in 2014 with a degree in English literature. In college he enjoyed reading timeless works of fiction and discussing them in the small classroom setting. He enjoyed writing and was passionate about storytelling and took several creative writing courses developing his own creative writing concentration of study. He graduated with College Honors and as a member of the English honor society. He discovered his calling to medicine during a summer internship before his senior year. He was working at a technology company that developed cloud-based medical records for hospitals. Working in the health care field helping to implement the technology, he was inspired by the work the doctors in the hospital do every day and realized he wanted to be helping patients directly. He saw medicine as a way he could help people—fusing his interest in the sciences and storytelling. After graduating from WashU, he decided to take the premedical courses required to apply to medical school. He enrolled in the 2-year postbaccalaureate program at New York University. After completing the program, he decided to join a cancer immunology research lab as a research assistant to help to develop new immunotherapeutic treatments for blood cancer. He contributed to several publications in peer reviewed medical journals in this area of research. He applied to medical school and decided to attend Albert Einstein College of Medicine in the Bronx, New York. He will be graduating with a distinction in research in May 2022. He lives in Hanover, NH with his wife, Rian, and their dog Bertie. He enjoys hiking throughout New England, hosting dinner parties, trail running, mountain biking, and playing basketball. He is starting internal medicine residency at Dartmouth in the summer of 2022.

Made in the USA
Middletown, DE
19 April 2022

64470574R00046